How To Get Rid Of Depression And Feel Happier

318 Great Tips To Beat Melancholy And Sadness

ADAM COLTON

Published by BizMove
www.bizmove.com

Table of Contents

1. Depression Fact Sheet

Depression (major depressive disorder or clinical depression) is a common but serious mood disorder. It causes severe symptoms that affect how you feel, think, and handle daily activities, such as sleeping, eating, or working. To be diagnosed with depression, the symptoms must be present for at least two weeks.

Some forms of depression are slightly different, or they may develop under unique circumstances, such as:

Persistent depressive disorder (also called dysthymia) is a depressed mood that lasts for at least two years. A person diagnosed with persistent depressive disorder may have episodes of major depression along with periods of less severe symptoms, but symptoms must last for two years to be considered persistent depressive disorder.

Perinatal depression is much more serious than the "baby blues" (relatively mild depressive and anxiety symptoms that typically clear within two weeks after delivery) that many women experience after giving birth. Women with perinatal depression experience full-blown major depression during pregnancy or after delivery (postpartum depression). The feelings of extreme sadness, anxiety, and exhaustion that accompany perinatal depression may make it difficult for these new mothers to complete daily care activities for themselves and/or for their babies.

Psychotic depression occurs when a person has severe depression plus some form of psychosis, such as having disturbing false fixed beliefs (delusions) or hearing or seeing upsetting things that others cannot hear or see (hallucinations). The psychotic symptoms typically have a depressive "theme," such as delusions of guilt, poverty, or illness.

Seasonal affective disorder is characterized by the onset of depression during the winter months, when there is less natural sunlight. This depression generally lifts during spring and summer. Winter depression, typically accompanied by social withdrawal, increased sleep, and weight gain, predictably returns every year in seasonal affective disorder.

Bipolar disorder is different from depression, but it is included in this list is because someone with bipolar disorder experiences episodes of extremely low moods that meet the criteria for major depression (called "bipolar depression"). But a person with bipolar disorder also experiences extreme high – euphoric or irritable – moods called "mania" or a less severe form called "hypomania."

Examples of other types of depressive disorders newly added to the diagnostic classification of <u>DSM-5</u> include disruptive mood dysregulation disorder (diagnosed in children and adolescents) and premenstrual dysphoric disorder (PMDD).

Signs and Symptoms

If you have been experiencing some of the following signs and symptoms most of the day, nearly every day, for at least two weeks, you may be suffering from depression:

- Persistent sad, anxious, or "empty" mood
- Feelings of hopelessness, or pessimism
- Irritability
- Feelings of guilt, worthlessness, or helplessness
- Loss of interest or pleasure in hobbies and activities

- Decreased energy or fatigue
- Moving or talking more slowly
- Feeling restless or having trouble sitting still
- Difficulty concentrating, remembering, or making decisions
- Difficulty sleeping, early-morning awakening, or oversleeping
- Appetite and/or weight changes
- Thoughts of death or suicide, or suicide attempts
- Aches or pains, headaches, cramps, or digestive problems without a clear physical cause and/or that do not ease even with treatment

Not everyone who is depressed experiences every symptom. Some people experience only a few symptoms while others may experience many. Several persistent symptoms in addition to low mood are required for a diagnosis of major depression, but people with only a few – but distressing – symptoms may benefit from treatment of their "subsyndromal" depression. The severity and frequency of symptoms and how long they last will vary depending on the individual and his or her particular illness. Symptoms may also vary depending on the stage of the illness.

Risk Factors

Depression is one of the most common mental disorders in the U.S. Current research suggests that depression is caused by a combination of genetic, biological, environmental, and psychological factors.

Depression can happen at any age, but often begins in adulthood. Depression is now recognized as occurring in children and adolescents, although it sometimes presents with more prominent irritability than low mood. Many chronic mood and anxiety disorders in adults begin as high levels of anxiety in children.

Depression, especially in midlife or older adults, can co-occur with other serious medical illnesses, such as diabetes, cancer, heart disease, and Parkinson's disease. These conditions are often worse when depression is present. Sometimes medications taken for these physical illnesses may cause side effects that contribute to depression. A doctor experienced in treating these complicated illnesses can help work out the best treatment strategy.

Risk factors include:

- Personal or family history of depression
- Major life changes, trauma, or stress
- Certain physical illnesses and medications

Treatment and Therapies

Depression, even the most severe cases, can be treated. The earlier that treatment can begin, the more effective it is. Depression is usually treated with <u>medications</u>, <u>psychotherapy</u>, or a combination of the two. If these treatments do not reduce symptoms, electroconvulsive therapy (ECT) and other brain stimulation therapies may be options to explore.

Quick Tip: No two people are affected the same way by depression and there is no "one-size-fits-all" for treatment. It may take some trial and error to find the treatment that works best for you.

Medications

Antidepressants are medicines that treat depression. They may help improve the way your brain uses certain chemicals that control mood or stress. You may need to try several different antidepressant medicines before finding the one that improves your symptoms and has manageable side effects. A medication that has helped you or a close family member in the past will often be considered.

Antidepressants take time – usually 2 to 4 weeks – to work, and often, symptoms such as sleep, appetite, and concentration problems improve before mood lifts, so it is important to give medication a chance before reaching a conclusion about its effectiveness. If you begin taking antidepressants, do not stop taking them without the help of a doctor. Sometimes people taking antidepressants feel better and then stop taking the medication on their own, and the depression returns. When you and your doctor have decided it is time to stop the medication, usually after a course of 6 to 12 months, the doctor will help you slowly and safely decrease your dose. Stopping them abruptly can cause withdrawal symptoms.

Please Note: In some cases, children, teenagers, and young adults under 25 may experience an increase in suicidal thoughts or behavior when taking antidepressants, especially in the first few weeks after starting or when the dose is changed. This warning from the U.S. Food and Drug Administration (FDA) also says that patients of all ages taking antidepressants should be watched closely, especially during the first few weeks of treatment.

If you are considering taking an antidepressant and you are pregnant, planning to become pregnant, or breastfeeding, talk to your doctor about any increased health risks to you or your unborn or nursing child.

You may have heard about an herbal medicine called St. John's wort. Although it is a top-selling botanical product, the FDA has not approved its use as an over-the-counter or prescription medicine for depression, and there are serious concerns about its safety (it should never be combined with a prescription antidepressant) and effectiveness. Do not use St. John's wort before talking to your health care provider. Other natural products sold as dietary supplements, including omega-3 fatty acids and S-adenosylmethionine (SAMe), remain under study but have not yet been proven safe and effective for routine use.

Psychotherapies

Several types of psychotherapy (also called "talk therapy" or, in a less specific form, counseling) can help people with depression. Examples of evidence-based approaches specific to the treatment of depression include cognitive-behavioral therapy (CBT), interpersonal therapy (IPT), and problem-solving therapy.

Brain Stimulation Therapies

If medications do not reduce the symptoms of depression, electroconvulsive therapy (ECT) may be an option to explore. Based on the latest research:

- ECT can provide relief for people with severe depression who have not been able to feel better with other treatments.

- Electroconvulsive therapy can be an effective treatment for depression. In some severe cases where a rapid response is necessary or medications cannot be used safely, ECT can even be a first-line intervention.

- Once strictly an inpatient procedure, today ECT is often performed on an outpatient basis. The treatment consists of a series of sessions, typically three times a week, for two to four weeks.

- ECT may cause some side effects, including confusion, disorientation, and memory loss. Usually these side effects are short-term, but sometimes memory problems can linger, especially for the months around the time of the treatment course. Advances in ECT devices and methods have made modern ECT safe and effective for the vast majority of patients. Talk to your doctor and make sure you understand the potential benefits and risks of the treatment before giving your informed consent to undergoing ECT.

- ECT is not painful, and you cannot feel the electrical impulses. Before ECT begins, a patient is put under brief anesthesia and given a muscle relaxant. Within one hour after the treatment session, which takes only a few minutes, the patient is awake and alert.

Other more recently introduced types of brain stimulation therapies used to treat medicine-resistant depression include repetitive transcranial magnetic stimulation (rTMS) and vagus nerve stimulation (VNS). Other types of brain stimulation treatments are under study.

If you think you may have depression, start by making an appointment to see your doctor or health care provider. This could be your primary care practitioner or a health provider who specializes in diagnosing and treating mental health conditions.

Beyond Treatment: Things You Can Do

Here are other tips that may help you or a loved one during treatment for depression:

- Try to be active and exercise.
- Set realistic goals for yourself.
- Try to spend time with other people and confide in a trusted friend or relative.
- Try not to isolate yourself, and let others help you.
- Expect your mood to improve gradually, not immediately.

- Postpone important decisions, such as getting married or divorced, or changing jobs until you feel better. Discuss decisions with others who know you well and have a more objective view of your situation.
- Continue to educate yourself about depression.

2. 318 Great Tips To Beat Melancholy And Sadness

If you can recognize the symptoms of depression and admit to yourself that you may be suffering from it, you have just taken the first step to beating this affliction. Once you overcome depression, you will find out what you've been missing in life. follow the following ideas and reach that level of happiness you feel is so elusive.

1. If you are trying to work on controlling your depression, get rid of unhealthy relationships. Many times, people who suffer from depression find their symptoms getting worse when they have people in their lives who put them down or discourage them from feeling better. Stay around positive and supportive people.

2. Make sure you're getting about eight hours of sleep a night. People with depression tend to either sleep too little or far too much. In either case, both your mood and your health will suffer. Schedule your sleep patterns so that you're getting just the right amount of sleep each night.

3. If you are suffering from depression, take a realistic account of your life now, as well as, your goals for the future. If you believe you 'can't be happy until' you have the ideal relationship, or higher income, or the like, then look at what is really important! Ask yourself if you "~it is really that bad now' or if you "~are setting reasonable goals.' If you are in a situation that is not likely to change, see if you can change the way you look at it.

4. One of the best ways to battle depression is to eat a healthy, well-balanced diet and avoid emotional eating. People often times tend to overeat as a way to escape their depression and avoid dealing with uncomfortable inner feelings. By overeating, you are only putting off feelings that need to be dealt with and, in the long run, making your depression worse.

5. If you have a good relationships with your family members then you should incorporate their help in overcoming your depression. Many times mothers and fathers are much more understanding than their children give them credit for. If you stop and tell them what is going on they will probably be happy to help.

6. Find an activity you enjoy such as a concert, time with friends who make you laugh or a funny movie. Sometimes that's all you need to feel better.

7. Do not blame yourself for your feelings of sadness when you have depression. Often times, people think that depression is their fault, when in fact, it is something that is beyond their control. The blame they put on themselves just ends up making their depression symptoms get worse and lowers their self esteem.

8. If you are the parent of a child or teenager and feel like they may have depression, it is important that you get them seen by a psychiatrist or therapist as soon as you can. When a child is treated for depression at a young age, they are more apt to live a productive life as an adult.

9. If your job is part of the cause of your depression, you may want to think of cutting down on some of your harder duties. Talk to your boss about how you are feeling and ask if you can do lighter projects. Try not to bring the stresses of your job home with you.

10. If you see a therapist for your depression, it is important that you are honest with them about

how you feel. By holding back or not telling your therapist the truth, you are preventing them from properly treating you. Remember, whatever you talk about with your therapist stays between the two of you.

11. If you do not get the results you want when you take one anti-depressant medication, speak to your doctor about trying another. People respond differently to various anti-depressants, and some work for some people and not for others. It may take some trial and error until you find the medication that works to relieve your depression.

12. A simple tip that is easy to do if you are depressed is to keep yourself clean and groomed. It is easy to sleep a lot and feel too lazy to take a shower when you are depressed. However, staying clean is important to remaining healthy and keeping your spirits high. Just the simple act of brushing your teeth or shaving will improve your mood. Within minutes, you will feel better.

13. Maintain social activities that you previously enjoyed, currently enjoy, or may not know much about. This can take your mind off of depressing matters that can send you back into your depression in a way that is worse than before.

You should surround yourself with social activities that are nurturing and can help stimulate your mind.

14. To assist with managing depression, examine your diet and what you are eating on a regular basis. Junk food is filled with preservatives and sugars which does not provide natural energy to the body. Fresh fruits and vegetables will give the body the nutrients and vibrancy needed to help focus on lifting your mood.

15. One way of dealing with depression is to practice using positive visualization. Start by closing your eyes and relaxing as much as possible. Take some deep breaths, and then begin imagining bright, happy scenes in your mind. For instance, if you love the outdoors you could visualize yourself sitting by a beautiful stream with birds singing in the trees nearby. By choosing happy, uplifting scenes and then vividly imagining them, you can instantly lift your mood and begin feeling better.

16. For some people, depression occurs during the winter months. Studies have shown that this is directly correlated to the amount of light that people are exposed to; in the absence of light, people's moods tended to be worse. Make the

most of the day during the winter by opening up your windows and going outside. Invest in white light bulbs (instead of fluorescent) to mimic natural light during the night.

17. As the beginning of this article told you, the first step to beating depression is admitting that you're suffering from it. The next step is to use what you've learned here to build a strategy to get over your mood disorder once and for all. It's doable, but you have to do it! It won't happen by itself.

18. Never stop a medication on your own. Many people will start a new medication when they are feeling down then immediately stop taking it when they are feeling better. This is a terrible idea as it can actually cause you to feel even worse than you did initially. Always consult a doctor before stopping.

19. Make sure that you avoid sugar, as this ingredient can worsen your depression upon consumption. Compared with complex carbohydrates, these simple sugars are absorbed more quickly into the bloodstream. This means that the person consuming the food will get a quick infusion of energy but will then feel tired and depressed later.

20. Go back to activities you used to enjoy, even if you don't feel like it. Going through the motions of a fun activity, such as painting or playing a sport, can help you feel more energetic. You might find that are truly enjoying the activity after all, once you get started.

21. Try to get outside as much as you can, when suffering from depression. Even if it is just for a quick walk every day, getting some sun and fresh air, can make a world of a difference for controlling depression symptoms. Sitting inside all the time, will just make you feel worse.

22. In order to help you manage your depression symptoms, you should aim to meditate regularly. Meditation is a proven method of lowering blood pressure and enhancing your mood.

23. If you have medical depression you should anticipate that many people won't be able to understand it. Most people think that depression is just like being really sad but true sufferers know that this is not the truth. If people say things like "just chin up" to you, try to realize that they mean the best and just ignore it.

24. Have realistic expectations. Often depressed people fixate on some unrealistic goal that they believe will cure their depression. For some it is money, for others it may be longing for an idealistic Mr. or Miss. "Right" to spend the rest of their life with. While having a goal is good, keep it realistic. Instead of being unhappy with your current job and longing to win the lottery, take college courses or a vocational program to increase your income potential. If you are lonely, get out and get involved with activities you enjoy. Even if you don't meet someone, you will have fun; and if you do meet someone, they are much more likely to have similar interests to you unlike a random stranger in a bar.

25. Examine your life. If you are unhappy because you feel like you are being walked on, focus on becoming more assertive. If you find yourself assuming people are thinking badly of you, remind yourself that you are not a mind-reader and that you have no basis for that belief. Keep it light and humorous, as you cannot battle negative thoughts with more negativity.

26. If you are a parent, and you start to feel a bout of depression coming on try to find a way for your children to not be around you. If they are older, you can leave them home alone, but if they

are younger children, you should have a close friend on standby to watch them.

27. Consider starting a depression diary. Get your feelings and thoughts down on paper can help you a bit feel better. Reflecting back on your journal can help you find what is triggering your depression most often.

28. If you are the family member or friend of someone who has depression, it is important that you are supportive. Your depressed loved ones needs reassurance and comfort during their difficult times. There are many resources to turn to, such as the internet and books, that can help guide you to be there for your loved one.

29. Keep a positive attitude. Negative thinking is always present in a person that has depression. Depressed people tend to minimize all of the good in their lives, while happy people keep a positive attitude by accepting sadness as a normal part of life, and fixing what they can. Being positive will also make you more pleasant to be around, and there is a lesser chance you will be lonely.

30. Clean your house, one room a day if necessary, when you feel depressed. It is normal to have

little or no motivation when depressed and this contributes to a messy house. This is a vicious cycle though, as a messy house can lead to more depression. Cleaning your house leads to an improved mood.

31. Try increasing your Vitamin B's intake to combat depression. Recent studies have shown a link between low levels of this vitamin and depression. Some of the best food sources of Vitamin B include meat, fish, poultry, eggs, fortified breakfast cereal and milk. You can also try taking a B-Complex Vitamin to be sure your are getting the recommended daily amount.

32. Pretend that you are happy. Many times, putting a fake smile on, and attempting to act and think happily can actually cause your mood to change. Faking these changes with your body actually increases the amount of happiness-inducing chemicals produced, which causes you to start to feel the happiness you are outwardly portraying.

33. Sleep is important when you are depressed. You will need to control the number of hours you allow yourself to sleep during the day and night. While getting the proper amount is required, it is also important not to get too much sleep as this can make matters worse rather than better.

34. A great tip that can help you out of depression is to force yourself to do the things you normally like to do. When we're depressed, we usually lose interest in all of our favorite activities. By forcing yourself to do your favorite activities, you'll be able to keep your spirits up.

35. If you are dealing with depression, slowly work on trying to fix some of the problems in your life. Many times, a difficult situation in your life is the reason for the depression in the first. Even if your depression wasn't caused by the issues in your personal life, an easier life will make it simpler to deal with the depression.

36. A good tip to help deal with depression is to develop some outside interests or hobbies. Those who suffer from depression need activities and events to look forward to. Try something you have always wanted to do, such as dancing, art or skydiving. While enjoying those activities, also develop new exciting interests.

37. Never underestimate the role of diet, exercise, and good sleep in staving off depression. If you are feeling depressed, a quick fix may be a swim, bike ride, run or brisk walk. In the long term, avoiding processed foods, getting light exercise

daily, and being certain to get 8 hours of good sleep every night may permanently chase away your blues.

38. Make sure you are getting enough Vitamin B in your diet if you suffer from depression. Having a deficiency of Vitamin B can cause depression symptoms to act up. Foods like leafy greens, beans, eggs, and chicken have Vitamin B. Also, there are supplements that you can take that contain this vitamin.

39. Know that you are not crazy. Depression is a real illness and should be afforded the same respect as any other disease. It is your body telling you that something is wrong, whether it is a chemical imbalance in the brain or unresolved emotions. Depression is your body's way of telling you that it is becoming overwhelmed and needs help.

40. Experiencing depression when you have a small child can be exceptionally difficult. This is because they are unlikely to understand why mommy or daddy is so sad all the time. While you don't want to hide your problem from them you also don't want to expose them to your negativity.

41. If you have real clinical depression do not
expect it to go away over night. This will be a
battle that you will have in your life for quite
some time to come. Because of this you should
start reading up now to prepare yourself for
some of the trials to come.

42. Come up with a positive phrase that you can
repeat to yourself whenever you start to feel
depressed. You need to combat the negative
thoughts by drowning them out with positive
thoughts. Even if you do not believe your
mantra, it will still help. You need to avoid letting
the negative feelings take over. Say your phrase
throughout the day, and eventually your mind
will start to think it is true.

43. Do not deny your emotions. For depression
caused by a traumatic event or loss, it is
important to let yourself feel the pain and
sadness. You should not dwell on it, however, it
is important to not bottle it away. It will only
surface later, and often in more harmful ways.

44. Depression comes in all shapes and sizes. The
first thing to realize about depression is that if
you have it, you don't need to be ashamed of it.
Seeking out professional help should never make
you feel like a failure or a weak person. It takes a

strong individual to realize and accept that they need help.

45. If you see a therapist for your depression, it is important that you are honest with them about how you feel. By holding back or not telling your therapist the truth, you are preventing them from properly treating you. Remember, whatever you talk about with your therapist stays between the two of you.

46. To assist with managing depression, examine your diet and what you are eating on a regular basis. Junk food is filled with preservatives and sugars which does not provide natural energy to the body. Fresh fruits and vegetables will give the body the nutrients and vibrancy needed to help focus on lifting your mood.

47. When it comes to managing your depression, be sure that you check with other people that you know and trust before making any life changing decisions. This is important so that you do not make any decisions that you cannot reverse while not in the best state of mind.

48. One way of dealing with depression is to practice using positive visualization. Start by closing your eyes and relaxing as much as

possible. Take some deep breaths, and then begin imagining bright, happy scenes in your mind. For instance, if you love the outdoors you could visualize yourself sitting by a beautiful stream with birds singing in the trees nearby. By choosing happy, uplifting scenes and then vividly imagining them, you can instantly lift your mood and begin feeling better.

49. A good tip that can help you get out of your depression is to not label yourself as someone that's depressed. If you're always telling yourself that you're in a depression, you'll most likely stay depressed. How can you expect to get better if you're always seeing yourself as so depressed?

50. Banish your blue moods by cutting sugar out of your diet, including the natural sugars contained in honey, fruits and molasses. Sugar will enter the bloodstream much quicker than the complex carbohydrate founds in whole grain products. This then causes a burst of energy, but then you have a "sugar crash" not too long after and a feeling of depression.

51. If you are trying to work on controlling your depression, get rid of unhealthy relationships. Many times, people who suffer from depression find their symptoms getting worse when they

have people in their lives who put them down or discourage them from feeling better. Stay around positive and supportive people.

52. Depression, which can be like a fog that isolates you from the rest of the world, is hard to lift and keep away by yourself. Getting supportive relationships can play a major role in beginning to defeat depression. Even though the nature of depression can make you want to retreat from others, remind yourself that your trusted friends and family members want to help. They can help lead you through this tough time in your life.

53. Consider taking a dietary supplement. Studies have shown that vitamin deficiencies can affect brain function, leading to disorders such as depression. Especially implicated are B vitamins, including folic acid and B-12. A chromium supplement, while not fixing a deficiency, will also help boost energy levels and reduce junk food cravings.

54. Eat a healthy diet. Many times someone who is depressed my try to cover those feelings with overeating, binge drinking, or even starving themselves. Suppressed feelings are one of the largest contributing factors in depression. When you find yourself reaching for the bag of cookies

or bottle of wine, remind yourself that you are making the feelings worse. In addition to forcing you to deal with your feelings instead of covering them, maintaining healthy eating habits will improve your health as well as your mood.

55. Reaching out to help other people can be a wonderfully effective way to overcome the challenges of depression that you may be facing yourself. With depression, there is often a tendency to focus inward and shut out the outside world. Making the effort to look past your own pain and help another person will remind you of the power you have to improve a life and influence activities in your own world. Look for opportunities to volunteer your services in your community and know that you will be expanding your opportunities to bring joy to yourself and those you reach out to help.

56. Try to pamper yourself if your depression symptoms are bothering you. Going to a salon to have your nails done or going to a spa to have a massage can help relax your mind and body and thus, reduce your depression symptoms. You may also want to buy yourself a special treat, like a shirt you have been wanting.

57. A simple tip that is easy to do if you are depressed is to keep yourself clean and groomed. It is easy to sleep a lot and feel too lazy to take a shower when you are depressed. However, staying clean is important to remaining healthy and keeping your spirits high. Just the simple act of brushing your teeth or shaving will improve your mood. Within minutes, you will feel better.

58. Consider joining a support group for people suffering from depression. Having a group of peers to talk to who are dealing with many of the same problems you are facing can be a tremendous asset. Additionally, being a part of a group can help reduce any feelings of isolation that you may be experiencing. By providing each other with support, encouragement and understanding, all of the members of your group can benefit.

59. Being more realistic about your expectations in life can help to alleviate your depression. A lot of times you may feel down because things are not turning out the way you had hoped or planned. If you examine the situation, you may often find that the real problem is that you had simply set your expectations unreachably high.

60. Surround yourself with beautiful things. When you can look around and see things that are beautiful and joyful, you, yourself, can feel more joy within and more positive as well. You will see just how easy it is to be happier when you can see pretty things all around you.

61. Keep your thoughts positive. This is easier said than done, because many times our minds automatically default to negative thoughts rather than positive ones. Try keeping track of your thoughts and putting your negativity into specific words. Sometimes, negative thoughts just want to be heard, and allowing them to exist gives them to freedom to dissipate.

62. Get plenty of sleep. Getting enough sleep leads to better health and refreshes your mind so you can fight off depression. When you're tired, depression and anxiety symptoms are much more prevalent. If you have insomnia, try to meditate before you go to bed, or get a sleeping aid.

63. Dress up. When you dress nicely, your mood improves. Making yourself look and feel attractive can help to show yourself that you have importance. Knowing that you are at your best can make your health and mood better, and

cause you to have a better outlook on life in general.

64. A great tip that can help you out of depression is to force yourself to do the things you normally like to do. When we're depressed, we usually lose interest in all of our favorite activities. By forcing yourself to do your favorite activities, you'll be able to keep your spirits up.

65. Exercise regularly if you suffer from depression. Exercising releases endorphins that stimulate mood and reduce stress. Exercising also has long-term health consequences that can reduce depression. For instance, eating too much sugar is known to worsen depression symptoms in some people. Overweight individuals also suffer worse depression symptoms on average.

66. If you are feeling depressed, and you have the means, consider adopting a pet. Even a small pet such as a rodent can give you the feeling that someone else depends on you each day. Having a pet is especially helpful for beating depression if you live alone, since it means you don't come home to an empty house.

67. Make sure to get a sufficient amount of sleep if you suffer from depression. Sleeping too little or

too much can effect your mood and the way that you think. Try to set a certain time to go to sleep every night and try to wake up at the same time everyday.

68. If you have medical depression you should anticipate that many people won't be able to understand it. Most people think that depression is just like being really sad but true sufferers know that this is not the truth. If people say things like "just chin up" to you, try to realize that they mean the best and just ignore it.

69. A support network is absolutely crucial in overcoming and even, in living with clinical depression. Some of the best support groups are now found online on websites known as forums. These are typically formed by other people who are experiencing the same thing that you are and will be able to give you better advice.

70. If depression is the only company you keep, you will keep yourself depressed! As hard as it may be to face the world or anyone in it when you are feeling depressed, seeing a friend or family member may be the best remedy. Even if it's just to take your mind off of your troubles temporarily, you will find the company of others can go a long way in making you feel better!

71. Drink a lot of water if you are feeling depressed. The body can survive for weeks without food, but without water our body and brain will begin to shut down. It is almost impossible to be happy when your body is dehydrated because your brain is not working properly. Try to drink filtered water when possible because many cities water have chemicals in them, and we do not know how this affects our brain.

72. Continue doing your everyday routines even if you do not feel like participating in these mundane tasks. It is important to stay in control of your life. Try to live like normal and keep doing the things that are familiar to you. If you stop doing these activities, it will be much harder to rise out of the depression and start doing them again.

73. If you have been feeling down, uninterested in things that make you happy, and are having trouble with sleep, this could be depression. Identifying depression is the first step in solving it. If you have had these feelings for more than two weeks, it is important that you see a psychiatrist as soon as possible.

74. Getting enough sleep - and the right kind of sleep - should be a critical focus for someone trying to overcome depression. Estimates are that more than 80% of people with depression have trouble getting enough sleep. Often, insomnia or a sleep disorder can be the culprit behind the onset of depression if a patient is not getting the restorative stages of deep sleep needed to feel refreshed and energized. Practicing good sleep hygiene can help to turn around many sleep issues, including going to bed at a set time, avoiding caffeine and alcohol in the evenings, and removing the television and other distractions from the bedroom. But when self-help methods don't resolve long term sleep issues, then seek help from a sleep expert or sleep clinic.

75. You may want to think about getting into aromatherapy if you suffer from depression. The natural fragrances help to stimulate the part of the brain that produces happiness and peace. Some oils, such as chamomile, basil, neroli, and damask rose, are especially helpful in treating feelings associated with depression.

76. Refrain from seeking to be perfect. No one is perfect, regardless of the image they portray or the feelings they give off. Even with all the

confidence in the world, perfection is a word for the Gods and you should always remember that you will have flaws, but it is these flaws that make you unique.

77. Develop and practice effective relaxation exercises or practices. Whether lying in a tub that is filled with aromatic beads or using Yoga to relax your mind, you want to keep a clear head and refrain from discomfort in order to avoid a depressed mood. With relaxation comes enlightenment and a much healthier mood.

78. Beat depression by developing your interests. Depression robs us by dampening our desire to pursue activities we used ot enjoy. Activities and various interests are critical to maintaining a happy, fulfilled frame of mind. Depression, worry, anger, anxiety and other negative emotions can be released through activities, especially if you do them whenever you feel bad.

79. Never stop a medication on your own. Many people will start a new medication when they are feeling down then immediately stop taking it when they are feeling better. This is a terrible idea as it can actually cause you to feel even worse than you did initially. Always consult a doctor before stopping.

80. One way to deal with depression is to "fake it till you make it". This means to act, walk, talk, and eat as if you were not depressed. If nothing else, faking it will mean that other things in your life are not neglected while you are depressed. At best, the behaviors will help re-route your brain and actually help cure your depression.

81. Challenge your depressive thinking patterns. If you are thinking something about yourself, consider if you'd ever make that statement about another person. If the answer is no, you're probably being overly hard on yourself. Try to reframe these types of thoughts in a more realistic and constructive manner by making statements that provide suggestions on how to fix the problem.

82. Be sure to discuss your depression with your partner. Involve your partner in your treatment efforts such as regular exercise and counseling. Working together in these endeavors will help bring you closer as a couple, and will also make your treatment plan more effective than if you were going it alone.

83. If you are opposed to taking prescription medications for depression, try St. John's Wort.

This natural, herbal remedy for depression can be very effective. It works in much the same way as Prozac by increasing the availability of mid-brain serotonin. This helps elevate your mood and alleviate your feelings of sorrow.

84. Stop rewarding bad behavior. Many times someone who is depressed will wallow in self-pity, allowing others to coddle them and take care of their responsibilities. Others abuse drugs, alcohol, sex, and food as a way to feel better temporarily. All of these behaviors do not help the depression in any way other than a temporary fix. Take away the rewards and the depressed person can focus on the root of the depression.

85. Examine your life. If you are unhappy because you feel like you are being walked on, focus on becoming more assertive. If you find yourself assuming people are thinking badly of you, remind yourself that you are not a mind-reader and that you have no basis for that belief. Keep it light and humorous, as you cannot battle negative thoughts with more negativity.

86. If you are trying to beat depression, it is helpful to join a support group for depression. Support groups offer encouragement from others who have experienced what you are going through.

You can also receive and give advice on techniques on coping with depression. Being with others who understand what you are experiencing helps reduce your sense of isolation.

87. The best way to beat depression and kick the blues is to become active and exercise. It is not a quick fix to the problem of depression but it is an ongoing way to make life better and gives you something to look forward too tomorrow. Not only does it release stress, but it makes a person feel better about themselves and gives you some control over your life.

88. Play dress up. Take the time in the morning to get yourself ready, even if you are not going anywhere. Putting on your good clothes, including shoes, can increase your confidence and your mood. Feeling sloppy and frumpy in old, stained clothes may be comfortable, but it does nothing for your mood.

89. Beware, although alcohol can feel like your best friend when you are fighting depression it actually may just be your enabler. If you feel yourself drawn to alcohol in your hardest moments - then you should avoid it completely!

Alcohol and depression are very close cousins and love to team up on the unsuspecting!

90. When you feel depressed, it is important to remember that there is always a light at the end of the tunnel. People with depression feel like their condition will never get better and they give up on their treatment. It is important to be patient and keep a positive attitude.

91. Smile at yourself in the mirror even if you are feeling depressed. The simple act of smiling can actually make you feel happier. You can also try laughing hysterically in a ridiculously fake laugh. After a while, that fake smile or fake laugh might turn into a real one once you start to feel silly enough about what you are doing.

92. A great way to deal with depression is to change your attire. It is true that the way you dress can often directly impact how you feel about yourself. Be sure that you always dress your best no matter what it is that you are doing and both you and others will have a more positive view about you.

93. Over indulging in food may seem to provide some immediate relief but in reality it will only lead to longer term disappointment and worsen

depression. What ever is making you depressed will not be remedied by eating so try and find some other way to comfort yourself, one that you will not feel guilty about later.

94. A good tip that can help you get out of your depression is to start keeping a daily journal. Keeping a daily journal can be a good way to just get your feelings out and to express yourself honestly. You can also refer back to it if you want.

95. Challenge your depressive thinking patterns. If you are thinking something about yourself, consider if you'd ever make that statement about another person. If the answer is no, you're probably being overly hard on yourself. Try to reframe these types of thoughts in a more realistic and constructive manner by making statements that provide suggestions on how to fix the problem.

96. Don't let your depression interfere with your normal life. Just as people who are having trouble with physical diseases shouldn't stop everything, neither should you stop your life just because you are suffering from this problem. Find ways to motivate yourself to get out of the

house and you may even find the your
depression greatly reduces.

97. One of the common things that makes people
depressed is their diet. Overeating, binge
drinking, and starving are all ways that people
use to suppress their feelings. Instead of doing
this, let those feelings out. The poor diet always
leads to other problems, so if it is recognized and
dealt with, it can be handled properly and not
lead to other problems in the future.

98. If you have a good relationships with your
family members then you should incorporate
their help in overcoming your depression. Many
times mothers and fathers are much more
understanding than their children give them
credit for. If you stop and tell them what is going
on they will probably be happy to help.

99. Getting an appropriate amount of sleep is also
another great way to battle depression. Clinical
studies have very reliably shown that both those
who over sleep and those that under sleep are
more prone to experience clinical depression. If
you can, you should have a set sleep schedule
which allows for seven or eight hours of sleep.

100.   Try to avoid being alone in your saddest moments. Whether you are talking to a trusted friend or just watching television with your spouse, being together with another person can often help you to feel as though you are not holding on to this entire problem yourself and this will alleviate some of the pain.

101.   Identify the reason for your depression! It can stem from a myriad of sources. Perhaps, it should be carefully analyzed by a professional. The most common causes of depression are circumstantial and clinical. Circumstantial is caused by difficult situations that are currently in the person's life, while clinical is caused by a chemical imbalance!

102.   Listening to music is a very good way to fend off depression, but if you are able to, playing music can be even more effective. The same holds true for all of the arts, being involved in them, even if you aren't that good, can be a great way to deal with hard times.

103.   A handy tip for depression sufferers is to eat a variety of healthy, energizing foods. Depression can be exacerbated by diets full of sugar and other empty calories. Choosing fresh, organic produce can help lift one's spirits and can

provide life-affirming nutrients that are vital for good, physical as well as mental health.

104.   Depression can affect the whole family, not just the sufferer. Children especially feel left out when mom or dad are feeling sad and unable to participate in family activities. Make sure you take some time to explain what's going on, and reassure your child that you and your doctor are working hard to find healing for you.

105.   Stay away from caffeine if you are experiencing severe depression. A small amount of caffeine is still healthy, but if you drink a lot of coffee chances are you are making your depression worse. If you are a big coffee or soda drinker, you may want to consider switching over to decaffeinated versions of your favorite beverages.

106.   When it comes to dealing with depression, try to get at least a few minutes of sunlight per day. This is important because not only is this visually soothing, but the effects of a moderate amount of ultra violet rays can actually have a positive effect on your overall mood.

107.   Get a hobby. One of the most common reasons people develop depression is because

they do not have enough interests to stay busy. Finding a hobby and developing an interest can help you to realize that you are good at something, and that others enjoy the same hobby that you do.

108.   Be realistic. Make sure you set attainable goals, expect reasonable outcomes, and prepare for the worst to happen. Adjust your expectations and priorities to actually suit your life, and work with that. Changing your outlook on your surroundings can easily change the moods you experience and the opinions you have concerning them.

109.   If you are feeling nervous and want to calm yourself down, you should introduce more complex carbohydrates into your diet. Studies have shown that complex carbohydrates can cause you to relax and help you to calm down, which is great when combating depression, anxiety and nervousness. However, make sure not to overeat.

110.   Work on resolving the problems in your life. This is subjective, because what one person sees as a problem may not bother someone else. Only you know what life issues cause you angst. Resolving problems does not need to involve

dramatic steps -- ease into it by starting a journal and writing out all your thoughts on each topic.

111.   Sometimes the most effective treatment for depression is to take the time to be thankful for what you have. Meditating on the positive aspects of your life is beneficial and will change your bad mood into a good mood. You will feel better once you remember that you are very fortunate. Be grateful for the food you eat and the house you live in. The basics of life are still a true privilege.

112.   Focus on foods that are good for you when battling depression. If you body does not have good things to draw on, then your body can not help you in the fight. Keep your body happy with items like fruits and vegetables. Stay far away from junk food and food that you overindulge in.

113.   If your income is low and you are suffering from depression, try and find free or low-cost social services that can help you. Local governments offer community counseling services to those with low incomes, especially those people who qualify for Medicaid. These community counseling centers can also provide

free samples of medication for those who can't afford to fill a prescription.

114.   If you are going the medication route to treat your depression, try a lot of different drugs before giving up. It is a little-known fact that people who have been helped by antidepressant medication had to try an average of four different drugs to find the one that worked for them.

115.   If you're dealing with depression, create a positive social circle. The more people you have in your life to support you, the better off you'll be when you are feeling down. In addition, having people who expect you to do things with them prevents you from staying home and wallowing.

116.   If you are facing depression at sub clinical levels you may want to try some over the counter remedies. For example grape juice and St. Johns wart have both been shown to have a positive impact on the mental welfare of their users. It is also cheaper than the more common prescription therapy.

117.   Although it is obvious that depression typically leads to dark thoughts, you should do

everything in your power to avoid letting yourself enter into these cycles. Once you start fantasizing about your own death or suicide it can be quite difficult to break out of the feedback loop that makes you more and more depressed.

118.   Reaching out to help other people can be a wonderfully effective way to overcome the challenges of depression that you may be facing yourself. With depression, there is often a tendency to focus inward and shut out the outside world. Making the effort to look past your own pain and help another person will remind you of the power you have to improve a life and influence activities in your own world. Look for opportunities to volunteer your services in your community and know that you will be expanding your opportunities to bring joy to yourself and those you reach out to help.

119.   Go on a long walk to enjoy nature. Sometimes a change of scenery can help us appreciate life. Watch the animals leading their lives. Pay attention to the small details and try to find the beauty in nature. Breathe in the fresh air, relax, and let your mind wander as you walk.

120.   Keep a positive attitude. Negative thinking is always present in a person that has depression. Depressed people tend to minimize all of the good in their lives, while happy people keep a positive attitude by accepting sadness as a normal part of life, and fixing what they can. Being positive will also make you more pleasant to be around, and there is a lesser chance you will be lonely.

121.   An important tip for dealing with stress is to expose yourself to new experiences. This is a healthy way to open yourself to possible new ways to cope as well as meet new people. A change of scenery can sometime be all that it takes to feel better.

122.   Refrain from any negative thoughts, and be sure and write then down when they do come into your mind. In this way, you can re-examine just why you have these thoughts, how they make you feel, and how to substitute these distorted thoughts with positive, happy ones. Only when you understand your negative thought patterns can you rediscover positive thinking.

123.   Get enough sleep, typically 8 hours per night, with a 6 hour minimum. There are many

studies that have concluded that sleep patterns have a lot to do with mood and behavior, and those that aren't getting enough sleep have a higher chance of becoming depressed. Rest is essential for the brain to function healthier, and you want to be sure that you aren't clouded by fatigue throughout the day.

124.   A good tip that can help you get out of your deep depression is to start feeling grateful. Feeling grateful about everything in your life will change the way you think. You'll stop complaining and you'll probably realize that you have a whole lot going on for you.

125.   Understand your mind. Depression is not a sign of insanity, rather it means something is not right. Depression is just a sign that something in your life is unbalanced. It could be something in yourself, your environment, or may include both. Knowing you are not crazy can really help you feel more positive about your life.

126.   Depression can seem never ending, but with the proper changes to your life, counseling and even medications if necessary, it will come to an end. You will emerge a happier and healthier you at some point. Keep your head up and try to

think positively about the future. Above all, don't give up.

127.   If your depression has been brought on by a specific event, then you suffer from supranational depression. A great way to help yourself combat this type of depression is with Ignatia Amara. This is a homeopathic remedy that comes from the Saing Ignatiur bean and it helps control your emotions during times of extreme grief or hysteria.

128.   Focus on foods that are good for you when battling depression. If you body does not have good things to draw on, then your body can not help you in the fight. Keep your body happy with items like fruits and vegetables. Stay far away from junk food and food that you overindulge in.

129.   A great tip that can help you battle depression is to think about seeing a therapist. Seeing a therapist can help because it allows you to get things off your chest. It also lets you talk to someone who won't judge you. Seeing a therapist can do wonders if you're depressed.

130.   Remember to keep a positive attitude. Studies show that people who are depressed

often minimize their talents and accomplishments, instead focusing on the negative aspects of their life. Take a page out of the classic children's novel Pollyanna" and make a game out of positivity. In the novel, Pollyanna forces herself to find something good about every situation, no matter how small it may seem.

131.   Although it is obvious that depression typically leads to dark thoughts, you should do everything in your power to avoid letting yourself enter into these cycles. Once you start fantasizing about your own death or suicide it can be quite difficult to break out of the feedback loop that makes you more and more depressed.

132.   If you are suffering from depression, one of the best thing you can do to improve the state of your mental health is to spend time with positive people. The people you surround yourself with have a huge impact on your thoughts and feelings. If you constantly spend time with negative people you will feel negative yourself. Thoughts and feelings are contagious so surround yourself with positive people.

133.   Try to avoid being alone in your saddest moments. Whether you are talking to a trusted

friend or just watching television with your spouse, being together with another person can often help you to feel as though you are not holding on to this entire problem yourself and this will alleviate some of the pain.

134.   Identify the reason for your depression! It can stem from a myriad of sources. Perhaps, it should be carefully analyzed by a professional. The most common causes of depression are circumstantial and clinical. Circumstantial is caused by difficult situations that are currently in the person's life, while clinical is caused by a chemical imbalance!

135.   A good way to eliminate some depression is to listen to motivational speakers. Don't try to do it all yourself, listen to others who can help inspire you and show you different ways to think positively. If you can immerse yourself in uplifting thoughts of others or read about their uplifting stories and inspirational activities, this can only help make you feel less depressed.

136.   If you are feeling depressed during the day try to stop what you are doing and go for a quick walk in the sun. Sunlight helps your body to release some chemicals that actually make you

feel much happier. This is also true for people who are naturally depressed.

137.   Smile at yourself in the mirror even if you are feeling depressed. The simple act of smiling can actually make you feel happier. You can also try laughing hysterically in a ridiculously fake laugh. After a while, that fake smile or fake laugh might turn into a real one once you start to feel silly enough about what you are doing.

138.   Refrain from any negative thoughts, and be sure and write then down when they do come into your mind. In this way, you can re-examine just why you have these thoughts, how they make you feel, and how to substitute these distorted thoughts with positive, happy ones. Only when you understand your negative thought patterns can you rediscover positive thinking.

139.   When it comes to dealing with depression be sure that you listen to others and take their feedback to heart. This is important because more often than not it will be other people that notice a difference in you before you do. Believe those who care for you and work with them to help yourself feel better.

140. A great tip that can help you get out of your depression is to start forgiving people who have wronged you. Carrying around grudges and ill will only fuels negativity. Learn to let it all go and move on. You might find yourself feeling better in no time.

141. A great tip that can help you crawl out of your depression is to try art therapy. Art therapy helps because it allows you to express your feelings in a creative way. Some people might find art therapy beneficial because it might help them express themselves more honestly.

142. People dealing with depression will benefit from avoiding alcohol completely. Alcohol depresses you more and studies show that it makes depression worse. If alcohol is a problem, get it out of the house, and consider attending an AA meeting.

143. An effective way to resolve and overcome depression is to create some realistic goals that you can achieve. These goals can be anything from learning to play an instrument or setting a fitness goal. By living a more goal oriented life, you will be able to focus more of your thoughts on things that are making your life better rather than the issues causing your depression.

Accomplishing your goals will also serve as a vital source for the self esteem and self confidence that you will need to overcome depression.

144.   Don't neglect your social outlets. It is understandable that your depressed mood makes you want to skip all those normal outings and activities. Eventually, you will want to be involved in your normal activities and you will have a good time. You want to make certain you maintain your normal activities. When you neglect what you should normally be doing, you can sometimes get discouraged and more depressed.

145.   One way to deal with depression is to "fake it till you make it". This means to act, walk, talk, and eat as if you were not depressed. If nothing else, faking it will mean that other things in your life are not neglected while you are depressed. At best, the behaviors will help re-route your brain and actually help cure your depression.

146.   Try to get outside as much as you can, when suffering from depression. Even if it is just for a quick walk every day, getting some sun and fresh air, can make a world of a difference for

controlling depression symptoms. Sitting inside all the time, will just make you feel worse.

147. Change the bad habits in your life that keep you depressed. Be ruthlessly honest with yourself as you try to identify what these habits are. Try using positive thinking, assertiveness skills, and problem solving skills to tackle these negative habits and thoughts. Try using humor to deal with life's problems too, instead of letting the negativity drown you.

148. Know that you are not crazy. Depression is a real illness and should be afforded the same respect as any other disease. It is your body telling you that something is wrong, whether it is a chemical imbalance in the brain or unresolved emotions. Depression is your body's way of telling you that it is becoming overwhelmed and needs help.

149. Although having a boyfriend or girlfriend may seem like the answer to all of your depression problems, it is not. It is very possible to have a healthy relationship even when you are depressed but you should not look at the relationship itself as the key or solution to your problems.

150.   A helpful tip for anyone suffering from depression is to make an effort to cut crying, complaining and lengthy discussions of sadness out of your daily routine. Constant expressions of unhappiness may cause those around you to attempt to provide a sympathetic ear, which may actually end up perpetuating the depressive cycle. By trying to remain positive, you will avoid sinking into a rut of self-pity.

151.   When struggling with depression, consider breaking up your routine. Experiencing the same routine, day after day, can become monotonous and eventually it will start to bring you down. Temporarily changing your routine can get you out of a rut and help to alleviate your depression. Try taking a day off from work and doing something you have never tried before.

152.   Eat healthy meals at least three times a day. Sometimes poor nutrition can exacerbate depression. Treat your body with respect and eat healthy foods even if you do not feel hungry. Try to eat at the same times of day so that your natural cycles will be in sync.

153.   Do something that you truly enjoyed doing when you were a child. As we grow up, we sometimes try to act like we are too mature for

certain fun activities. If you loved swinging on a playground or playing board games, feel free to let your inner-child out and do those things.

154.   If you are actively trying to combat depression, know you are not alone. Studies have shown that everyone experiences depression at some point in their life. Take note that depression is real and must be treated proactively. If you are experiencing a difficult time, and you think you may be depressed, you probably are. Find ways to treat the depression yourself or seek professional help to get your life back on track.

155.   If you have children and you suffer from depression, it is important that you do not let them see that you are suffering. Children feed off of their parents words and actions and by them seeing you in a depressed condition, they may start to get feelings of depression themselves.

156.   When suffering from depression, sometimes it pays to forgive people who have done you wrong. Holding on to grudges and feeling hatred toward people can make you feel worse. Letting go of these negative feelings can help you learn how to feel more positive both toward yourself and toward others.

157.   To cure depression, you need to focus on being active. Exercise releases endorphins, which will naturally make you feel good. Don't think of this as a quick fix, but something you should be doing every day. If you think of being active as a life style, you will be much less likely to give up.

158.   Develop a routine. Having an established routine can help lessen depression by keeping unwelcome surprises out of your life. Knowing what to expect in your life can help you feel better and more prepared to deal with any unexpected events. Having a good schedule and a back-up plan are great methods of preparation.

159.   One of the fundamental ways to combat depression is to find interests and hobbies that you can involve yourself in. Interests and hobbies provide a way for you to keep your mind off the problems and issues that are causing your depression. Focusing on activities that you enjoy doing will also raise your overall happiness. If you are depressed, find something that you enjoy doing and commit time to it!

160.   Simple changes in lifestyle can help with depression. One way to make a dent in your depression is to exercise each day. Depression

can cause you to not have much energy, but just a short walk down the block and back can help you start becoming more energized. The road to recovering from depression requires taking pro-active measures.

161.   Be sure you are getting enough exercise every day. Studies have shown that people who get approximately thirty minutes of exercise a day respond better to depression treatment. In fact, exercise can be as powerful as a pharmaceutical anti-depressant. Simply taking the stairs or parking your car a little further from the store can benefit your physical and mental health.

162.   Be sure to discuss your depression with your partner. Involve your partner in your treatment efforts such as regular exercise and counseling. Working together in these endeavors will help bring you closer as a couple, and will also make your treatment plan more effective than if you were going it alone.

163.   By taking a hot bath, you can relieve depression and calm your nerves. Sitting in the bathtub reading your favorite novel or listening to a beloved album is a great way to relax and

make yourself feel great. Keep the water nice and warm as you soak, as this helps to relax muscles.

164.   A key tip in dealing with depression is to remember that you are the one in control of your own thoughts. Do not even use the word depressed as part of your vocabulary. It is a terrible way to describe how you're feeling, and it can have a negative effect on your state of mind. Use a neutral word or phrase instead, and focus on moving forward with positive thoughts and words.

165.   Although depression is often temporary, there are many cases where it can last for a lifetime. Because of this fact, you must learn how to live a fulfilling life, even when you are feeling depressed. This will entail different things for different people, but the key idea is to live normally.

166.   When depression hits, take the time to count your blessings. No matter if you are sad, or possibly angry, be thankful for what you do have and what you have going for you. There are people in this world who would gladly exchange their place for yours and not take the gifts that you have been given for granted. With a gracious

attitude and positive thoughts, depression cannot survive.

167.   A helpful tip for anyone suffering from depression is to make an effort to cut crying, complaining and lengthy discussions of sadness out of your daily routine. Constant expressions of unhappiness may cause those around you to attempt to provide a sympathetic ear, which may actually end up perpetuating the depressive cycle. By trying to remain positive, you will avoid sinking into a rut of self-pity.

168.   If you suffer from depression, try taking up a hobby. Interest in a new activity can take your mind off your daily troubles, as well as, provide some fun entertainment. Scrapbooking, photography, even painting can provide an outlet for your emotions and show off your creative skills!

169.   When it comes to depression consider seeking the help of professionals in order to help you. This is important to consider because you cannot always control everything in your life and you might not be able to fix everything yourself. Consider visiting a professional in order to get your life straightened out.

170.   One basic way to reduce depression is to get horizontal and have sex. Sex is known to release endorphins and when we are faced with long term depressing situations, we tend to forget about it and ignore our needs as human beings. Sex is one of the best all around total body relaxers and a great way to feel good about yourself.

171.   A good tip that can help you get out of your depression is to start keeping a daily journal. Keeping a daily journal can be a good way to just get your feelings out and to express yourself honestly. You can also refer back to it if you want.

172.   People feel depressed because they do not have any outside activities or interests. If your life has become boring and routine, try cultivating some interests. Try visiting the elderly, working with your hands or doing some house work. Having other interests can help you to feel better about yourself and increase your happiness.

173.   A great tip that can help you out of your depression is to see any dilemmas with a humorous perspective. A little humor can go a long way and can usually help you deal with a

very difficult situation. Use humor to help you get out of your depression.

174.   Stop for a couple of minutes each day to examine your blessings. Take the time to remember why it is you do the things you do in your life. The people and way of life that are important to you are the things that should motivate you. Touch on why each blessing in your life is important to you and let some of your negative feelings wash away.

175.   Keep a log of all your negative thoughts. Every time you notice a negative thought creeping up, write it down, and also write down what triggered you to have that thought. You can then look at it later and come up with better ways of dealing with the situation and find out if your negativity was really needed.

176.   Sometimes, a pet can be the one to help someone get over depression because they give you that feeling of being needed and loved. This can be exactly what someone suffering from depression needs. They can also make you get outside of yourself which is a great antidote for someone that is depressed.

177.   Remember to keep a positive attitude. Studies show that people who are depressed often minimize their talents and accomplishments, instead focusing on the negative aspects of their life. Take a page out of the classic children's novel Pollyanna" and make a game out of positivity. In the novel, Pollyanna forces herself to find something good about every situation, no matter how small it may seem.

178.   Be sure to discuss your depression with your partner. Involve your partner in your treatment efforts such as regular exercise and counseling. Working together in these endeavors will help bring you closer as a couple, and will also make your treatment plan more effective than if you were going it alone.

179.   When you feel your depression symptoms acting up, take a long bath. Listening to music or reading a beloved book in the tub can be a great mood-lifter. Make sure you use warm water; this will help your muscles get relaxed.

180.   Always think of depression as you would any other disorder or disease because that is exactly what it is. You don't need to hide it from the world and you should be sure to get medical

assistance if you feel the depression is lasting longer than a normal amount of sadness.

181. When suffering from depression, it is important to create a positive social life. Depressed individuals should work to make their social interactions more positive by showing kindness towards others and taking an interest in other people's lives. Depressed people should tell their friends and loved ones to ignore their depressed behaviors and not take pity on them.

182. If you have medical depression you should anticipate that many people won't be able to understand it. Most people think that depression is just like being really sad but true sufferers know that this is not the truth. If people say things like "just chin up" to you, try to realize that they mean the best and just ignore it.

183. Have realistic expectations. Often depressed people fixate on some unrealistic goal that they believe will cure their depression. For some it is money, for others it may be longing for an idealistic Mr. or Miss. "Right" to spend the rest of their life with. While having a goal is good, keep it realistic. Instead of being unhappy with your current job and longing to win the lottery, take college courses or a vocational program to

increase your income potential. If you are lonely, get out and get involved with activities you enjoy. Even if you don't meet someone, you will have fun; and if you do meet someone, they are much more likely to have similar interests to you unlike a random stranger in a bar.

184.   Drink a lot of water if you are feeling depressed. The body can survive for weeks without food, but without water our body and brain will begin to shut down. It is almost impossible to be happy when your body is dehydrated because your brain is not working properly. Try to drink filtered water when possible because many cities water have chemicals in them, and we do not know how this affects our brain.

185.   See your doctor. Not only is depression a real disease on its own, it can also be a symptom of other underlying illnesses. Only your doctor will be able to tell you what type of depression you are suffering from or if your symptoms are caused by another ailment. In addition, while many forms of depression can be treated without medication, it can also be caused by a chemical imbalance in the brain necessitating the use of medication for effective treatment.

186.   Take your prescribed medication the same time each day; the morning is preferred. If you follow a pattern, you should be less likely to forget your medication. Also, by taking the medication in the morning, this allows you to function normally through work, and also through your other daily responsibilities.

187.   When it comes to depression consider seeking the help of professionals in order to help you. This is important to consider because you cannot always control everything in your life and you might not be able to fix everything yourself. Consider visiting a professional in order to get your life straightened out.

188.   A great way to deal with depression is to make sure that you do not lose track of your social life. This is extremely important because if you do not have a social life, you may lose touch with the people who are in the best situation to help you with your problems.

189.   A great way to deal with depression is to change your attire. It is true that the way you dress can often directly impact how you feel about yourself. Be sure that you always dress your best no matter what it is that you are doing

and both you and others will have a more positive view about you.

190.   Maintain social activities that you previously enjoyed, currently enjoy, or may not know much about. This can take your mind off of depressing matters that can send you back into your depression in a way that is worse than before. You should surround yourself with social activities that are nurturing and can help stimulate your mind.

191.   Become more physically active. A healthy body is a necessity for a healthy mind. In addition to the obvious health benefits, exercising releases feel-good chemicals called endorphins. It is these chemicals that give rise to the term "runner's high". It is a natural high, one that is safe and even healthy to become addicted to!

192.   If you are trying to beat depression, it is helpful to join a support group for depression. Support groups offer encouragement from others who have experienced what you are going through. You can also receive and give advice on techniques on coping with depression. Being with others who understand what you are

experiencing helps reduce your sense of isolation.

193.   The best way to beat depression and kick the blues is to become active and exercise. It is not a quick fix to the problem of depression but it is an ongoing way to make life better and gives you something to look forward too tomorrow. Not only does it release stress, but it makes a person feel better about themselves and gives you some control over your life.

194.   Try to pamper yourself if your depression symptoms are bothering you. Going to a salon to have your nails done or going to a spa to have a massage can help relax your mind and body and thus, reduce your depression symptoms. You may also want to buy yourself a special treat, like a shirt you have been wanting.

195.   Get dancing! Exercise is good for depression, but getting the motivation for a workout is hard enough when you are not depressed. Instead, throw on your favorite upbeat music. No slow, depressing songs allowed. Close your curtains if you are shy, and let loose. Not only will the movement get your blood pumping, the music can lift your mood.

196.   A helpful tip for anyone suffering from depression is to make an effort to cut crying, complaining and lengthy discussions of sadness out of your daily routine. Constant expressions of unhappiness may cause those around you to attempt to provide a sympathetic ear, which may actually end up perpetuating the depressive cycle. By trying to remain positive, you will avoid sinking into a rut of self-pity.

197.   Acknowledging to yourself that your depression needs to be managed is a positive step. To avoid the temptation of sleeping in late or staying in bed throughout the day, purposely schedule appointments before noon to get you up and ready for the day. Always try to schedule your appointments early. Waiting until you wake up to decide your schedule, may put you at a disadvantage to taking charge of how you spend your day and you may be tempted to remain in bed because of the depression.

198.   Try aromatherapy as a treatment for depression. Certain scents are known to affect your mood. You can either buy ready-to-use aromatherapy oils or make your own. Simply dilute the herbs with a little vegetable oil and rub into your skin. You can also add a few drops to your bath water or scent the entire room with a

diffuser. Helpful herbs for depression include lavender, lemon, rose, and geranium.

199.   Sometimes it is the simple steps that help manage depression effectively. Writing lists of things to do is a great strategy because depression affects a person's ability to manage simple tasks without being overwhelmed. Writing down errands, goals or appointments will help keep peace of mind, and take the clutter out of your thoughts.

200.   Depression may cause a loss of appetite, but your body needs those nutrients to recover, so never starve yourself. Loss of appetite is a common symptom of depression. Even if you don't feel like eating, your body still needs nutrients.

201.   Developing interest will help you beat depression. Many people fall into a depression because they don't have anything they really enjoy doing. Having interests and activities that you find enjoyable are very important to your mental health and can raise your self-esteem as well as your happiness. These activities tend to bring a sense of satisfaction as well as keep your mind off anything negative in your life.

202.   If you find yourself suffering from intense depression, you should refrain from drinking caffeinated beverages. Studies have shown that too much caffeine can actually make depression worse. If you are a big coffee or soda drinker, you may want to consider switching over to decaffeinated versions of your favorite beverages.

203.   When suffering from depression, sometimes it pays to forgive people who have done you wrong. Holding on to grudges and feeling hatred toward people can make you feel worse. Letting go of these negative feelings can help you learn how to feel more positive both toward yourself and toward others.

204.   Develop and practice effective relaxation exercises or practices. Whether lying in a tub that is filled with aromatic beads or using Yoga to relax your mind, you want to keep a clear head and refrain from discomfort in order to avoid a depressed mood. With relaxation comes enlightenment and a much healthier mood.

205.   Be realistic. Make sure you set attainable goals, expect reasonable outcomes, and prepare for the worst to happen. Adjust your expectations and priorities to actually suit your

life, and work with that. Changing your outlook on your surroundings can easily change the moods you experience and the opinions you have concerning them.

206.   If you are trying to work on controlling your depression, get rid of unhealthy relationships. Many times, people who suffer from depression find their symptoms getting worse when they have people in their lives who put them down or discourage them from feeling better. Stay around positive and supportive people.

207.   Depression is something we all have faced at some point. If you are having bouts with depression you should see a psychologist. Often times, they can identify a problem in your way of thinking and work to reform it. In this way, the cause is treated and not just the symptoms.

208.   If you work on the personal problems that you are up against, this will help with your depression. Take small steps to avoid becoming overwhelmed and take on tasks one or two at a time. Breaking them into smaller goals will help combat depression and will probably fix many of the problems that are at the root cause of the depression.

209.   Become more physically active. A healthy body is a necessity for a healthy mind. In addition to the obvious health benefits, exercising releases feel-good chemicals called endorphins. It is these chemicals that give rise to the term "runner's high". It is a natural high, one that is safe and even healthy to become addicted to!

210.   Eat food that will make you feel positive about yourself. Eating lifeless and fatty fast food will make you not only look bad, but feel bad too. Do not think that the food that you eat has nothing to do with the way you feel and why you are depressed. Even if you crave the sugar or fat, these kinds of foods only lead to making you feel worse.

211.   Drink a lot of water if you are feeling depressed. The body can survive for weeks without food, but without water our body and brain will begin to shut down. It is almost impossible to be happy when your body is dehydrated because your brain is not working properly. Try to drink filtered water when possible because many cities water have chemicals in them, and we do not know how this affects our brain.

212.   If you are struggling with depression and low self-esteem, one of the best things you can do for your mental health is to spend time interacting with animals and nature. Animals show unconditional love and live life in the moment. Spending time with animals is a great way to help you improve your mood.

213.   Becoming interested in the arts is a great way to help you beat your depression. If you like paintings or sculpture be sure to schedule lots of visits to local museums. Likewise if you like music be sure to visit as many concerts and shows as you are able to.

214.   One of the best things depressed people can do is to learn gratitude. Being thankful for the positive things that you have in your life, in comparison to those that are less fortunate, will make you appreciate what you have, instead of dwelling on the things that you don't have.

215.   Try aromatherapy as a treatment for depression. Certain scents are known to affect your mood. You can either buy ready-to-use aromatherapy oils or make your own. Simply dilute the herbs with a little vegetable oil and rub into your skin. You can also add a few drops to your bath water or scent the entire room with a

diffuser. Helpful herbs for depression include lavender, lemon, rose, and geranium.

216.   For those who suffer from depression, get your spouse or partner to do the housework. It is important that you relax and avoid activities that could make your depression worse. If you feel bad about putting all of the responsibilities on to your spouse, offer to do the housecleaning one week and ask them to do it the next.

217.   If you suffer from depression, try to avoid a diet with lots of carbohydrates. Studies have shown that too many carbohydrates can cause depression or make it worse. Instead, try to eat a diet that has a lot of protein in it and try to eat a lot of fruits and vegetables.

218.   Consider joining a support group for people suffering from depression. Having a group of peers to talk to who are dealing with many of the same problems you are facing can be a tremendous asset. Additionally, being a part of a group can help reduce any feelings of isolation that you may be experiencing. By providing each other with support, encouragement and understanding, all of the members of your group can benefit.

219.   Surround yourself with beautiful things. When you can look around and see things that are beautiful and joyful, you, yourself, can feel more joy within and more positive as well. You will see just how easy it is to be happier when you can see pretty things all around you.

220.   One method to help battle depression is to choose to do activities that you used to enjoy. Even when you do not feel like it, push yourself to get out and do things. Surprisingly, you might feel a bit better once you are out and about. Do not be dismayed if your depression does not lift immediately. It is more common to gradually feel more upbeat after several efforts of making time for mood-boosting activities.

221.   If you suffer from depression you may want to consider getting a pet. The main part of depression is the feeling of loneliness and caring for a pet can help eliminate those feelings or isolation. Also, studies have shown that pet owners are less likely to feel depressed than people who do not have pets.

222.   One way to treat depression is with prescription medication. Every year new ones come out too, so if you tried one years ago there are many alternatives now. Most of them work

by attempting to restore the chemical balance in your brain as they believe depression is caused by a chemical imbalance.

223.   It is important to remember that no one is perfect. Many people who suffer from depression started the downward spiral because of thinking that just because they do not always do or say the right thing, there is something wrong with them. Focus on the qualities about yourself that you and everyone else admires. Yes, focus on your good points and use these to form a positive opinion of your overall self. This simple step can help you on the road to recovery.

224.   A simple walk around your block can be a wonderful mood elevator and a way to get those happy endorphins working to your advantage. If you have forgotten the joy of walking, then take your dog (or borrow one from a neighbor) and focus on his joy and antics for a few minutes. Getting out in your neighborhood keeps you in touch with what is going on around you and helps you take the focus off yourself for awhile.

225.   Make sure you are getting enough Vitamin B in your diet if you suffer from depression. Having a deficiency of Vitamin B can cause depression symptoms to act up. Foods like leafy

greens, beans, eggs, and chicken have Vitamin B. Also, there are supplements that you can take that contain this vitamin.

226.   Because of the possibility that your depression is caused by a chemical imbalance, some antidepressant drugs can work wonders. However, if you want normalcy restored in your life, you must also exercise and take part in therapy.

227.   The best way to beat depression and kick the blues is to become active and exercise. It is not a quick fix to the problem of depression but it is an ongoing way to make life better and gives you something to look forward too tomorrow. Not only does it release stress, but it makes a person feel better about themselves and gives you some control over your life.

228.   If you have a good relationships with your family members then you should incorporate their help in overcoming your depression. Many times mothers and fathers are much more understanding than their children give them credit for. If you stop and tell them what is going on they will probably be happy to help.

229.   Depression can have many root causes, and you should do your best to try and figure out what is the root of your personal depression. With the help of a doctor or therapist, you can begin to understand these feelings, and find treatment to help you cope with them.

230.   Identify the reason for your depression! It can stem from a myriad of sources. Perhaps, it should be carefully analyzed by a professional. The most common causes of depression are circumstantial and clinical. Circumstantial is caused by difficult situations that are currently in the person's life, while clinical is caused by a chemical imbalance!

231.   If you feel like your depression is reaching critical levels it may be time to get a change of scenery. Look at what is happening in your life and try to set a near date for a nice vacation. Even a weekend getaway is a great way to help change your thoughts.

232.   When struggling with depression, consider breaking up your routine. Experiencing the same routine, day after day, can become monotonous and eventually it will start to bring you down. Temporarily changing your routine can get you out of a rut and help to alleviate your depression.

Try taking a day off from work and doing something you have never tried before.

233.   If you feel like committing suicide or hurting someone else, it is important that you seek help immediately. These are signs that your depression has gotten out of control and you should get help before it is too late. Do not be scared to tell a professional if you are feeling this way.

234.   If you suffer from depression, try to avoid a diet with lots of carbohydrates. Studies have shown that too many carbohydrates can cause depression or make it worse. Instead, try to eat a diet that has a lot of protein in it and try to eat a lot of fruits and vegetables.

235.   When battling depression, it is important to keep stress in check. Stress will not only prolong depression, it will also make it worse. You need to examine your life and determine what is stressing you out. Once you have determined what are the main stressors in your life, you can develop a plan to minimize their impact or, if possible, avoid them altogether.

236.   Being realistic is one of the key things to do to overcome depression. Think about the things

you want to accomplish, and what you expect to receive from life. If they are not realistic, adjust your goals and your outlook. Having priorities that are impossible to achieve is just going to lead to failure, which will cause you to become more depressed once you fail to accomplish them.

237.   If you are the social type, then consider joining a depression support group. Depression support groups offer two things. The most important is a safe space to share stories and learn that you are not alone. Support groups are also a great place to learn practical tips for mitigating symptoms.

238.   Depression is something we all have faced at some point. If you are having bouts with depression you should see a psychologist. Often times, they can identify a problem in your way of thinking and work to reform it. In this way, the cause is treated and not just the symptoms.

239.   One way to treat depression is with prescription medication. Every year new ones come out too, so if you tried one years ago there are many alternatives now. Most of them work by attempting to restore the chemical balance in

your brain as they believe depression is caused by
a chemical imbalance.

240.   Don't be afraid to get help when you need it.
The perfectionist thinking that goes along with
depression, can often drive people to think that
seeing a therapist for depression is a sign of
weakness. But in fact, it's just the opposite.
Seeing a therapist means you're facing the
problem head-on and seeking a solution.

241.   To help you conquer your depression it is
vital that you learn to develop a positive attitude
and change the way you think. Research has
shown that negative thinking plays a huge role in
depression. Depressed people minimize their
successes and accomplishments and, instead,
focus on their failures and sorrows. The key to
happiness is loving life in the face of suffering.

242.   Play dress up. Take the time in the morning
to get yourself ready, even if you are not going
anywhere. Putting on your good clothes,
including shoes, can increase your confidence
and your mood. Feeling sloppy and frumpy in
old, stained clothes may be comfortable, but it
does nothing for your mood.

243.   Know that you are not crazy. Depression is a real illness and should be afforded the same respect as any other disease. It is your body telling you that something is wrong, whether it is a chemical imbalance in the brain or unresolved emotions. Depression is your body's way of telling you that it is becoming overwhelmed and needs help.

244.   Eat a healthy diet. Many times someone who is depressed my try to cover those feelings with overeating, binge drinking, or even starving themselves. Suppressed feelings are one of the largest contributing factors in depression. When you find yourself reaching for the bag of cookies or bottle of wine, remind yourself that you are making the feelings worse. In addition to forcing you to deal with your feelings instead of covering them, maintaining healthy eating habits will improve your health as well as your mood.

245.   To reduce depression, wear your favorite outfit or dress. Put on your best outfit and head out. Dress up for no other reason than to look amazing and boost your self esteem. By reminding yourself of how nice you can look and how attractive you can feel, you can boost your self-esteem, and perhaps lift your depression.

246.   Come up with a positive phrase that you can repeat to yourself whenever you start to feel depressed. You need to combat the negative thoughts by drowning them out with positive thoughts. Even if you do not believe your mantra, it will still help. You need to avoid letting the negative feelings take over. Say your phrase throughout the day, and eventually your mind will start to think it is true.

247.   Keep your friends and family close. Many people are willing to help you deal with your depression. Allow them into your life and include them in your situation. You will be surprised how understanding people are. Connecting with others in any way will only be beneficial to you and they might even be able to provide a few smiles.

248.   If you have begun taking medication for depression, do not be alarmed if you do not feel better right away. In fact, you may even feel worse when your medication does not work because you are nervous. Most anti-depressants take at least three weeks to settle into your system and help your symptoms.

249.   Being alone is not the solution to beating depression. Many people feel like being by

themselves when they are depressed, which just gives them the time to sit and dwell on negative things. If you do not feel like being around a large crowd, have your best friend come over to watch a movie.

250.   When your depression starts to act up, make sure you are eating and not starving yourself. People who are depressed may not eat sometimes because they are feeling upset. Even if you aren't a big eater, it is important to eat so your body continues to get the healthy nutrients it needs.

251.   A great way to deal with depression is to make sure that you do not lose track of your social life. This is extremely important because if you do not have a social life, you may lose touch with the people who are in the best situation to help you with your problems.

252.   When suffering from depression, sometimes it pays to forgive people who have done you wrong. Holding on to grudges and feeling hatred toward people can make you feel worse. Letting go of these negative feelings can help you learn how to feel more positive both toward yourself and toward others.

253.   Treat yourself with compassion. Have you ever seen someone yell at themselves when they make a mistake? Ever thrown a golf club after a bad swing? Being so hard on yourself can push you deeper down the depression spiral. Treat yourself with love and compassion, like you would treat a friend or a small child. Remind yourself that everyone makes mistakes, and that we all learn more from our failures than our successes.

254.   A great tip that can help you out of depression is to force yourself to do the things you normally like to do. When we're depressed, we usually lose interest in all of our favorite activities. By forcing yourself to do your favorite activities, you'll be able to keep your spirits up.

255.   If you are struggling with depression try not to get yourself caught up in the destructive mindset that the world is out to get you. This will only make you despair more and can do nothing but make your depression even worse and deeper than it was in the first place.

256.   Avoid using the words "depressed" or "depression." While depression is a tangible problem, the terminology that comes along with it can leave people feeling stigmatized and

overwhelmed. Rather, when feeling down, position it for yourself that you are in a low mood period. It is much easier to think about raising your mood level than it is to think of it as battling "depression", even though it is exactly what you are doing.

257.   One way to deal with depression is to fake it till you make it. Try to act as though you are not depressed. Really give it a good try and force yourself too. Imagine that you are not depressed and eventually it will come to pass. Basically you are tricking your mind, because if you do it enough, your brain will not know that it is depressed.

258.   You should never let yourself feel like a broken person because you are dealing with depression. Just as some people have to deal with bad lungs or a difficult disease, you have to deal with your depression. You should consider it to be nothing more than a nuisance in your life.

259.   Even something as simple and fresh flowers can brighten your home and mood. The smells and colors of flowers are very pleasant. So, use this to your advantage and pick up some fresh flowers.

260.   The best tip anyone could offer to someone who is depressed is to not make any big or rash decisions. Often times when we are depressed we make irrational decisions based on emotions not knowledge which often makes things worse. As such sit idly on those big decisions till you feel better.

261.   If your depression is flaring up during the winter months, you may want to consider taking a vacation to a warm climate. Winter flares up depression symptoms because people are stuck in their house more often. A relaxing vacation on the beach may help you feel better and help your depression.

262.   Stay away from energy drinks when you are feeling depressed. Although they may give you the energy you need because you are not sleeping enough, it is only a temporary relief. Instead, try more natural approached to help you sleep, such as listening to classical music or drinking a glass of mile before bed.

263.   A great way to deal with depression is to change your attire. It is true that the way you dress can often directly impact how you feel about yourself. Be sure that you always dress

your best no matter what it is that you are doing
and both you and others will have a more
positive view about you.

264.   Stick to a positive group of peers to combat
your depression. You will find that it is difficult
to remain in a depressed state when those
around you are bubbly and positive. Those who
are positive can even direct you into more
positive thinking patterns that help support a
more positive you.

265.   A good tip that can help you get out of your
deep depression is to start feeling grateful.
Feeling grateful about everything in your life will
change the way you think. You'll stop
complaining and you'll probably realize that you
have a whole lot going on for you.

266.   Depression can be especially crippling when
it happens to someone around you. You should
observe the person who is depressed, in order to
better understand why they are depressed.
Sometimes this can lead to beneficial results such
as observing their diet and seeing if perhaps
there is a biochemical imbalance in their diet.

267.   Understand your mind. Depression is not a
sign of insanity, rather it means something is not

right. Depression is just a sign that something in your life is unbalanced. It could be something in yourself, your environment, or may include both. Knowing you are not crazy can really help you feel more positive about your life.

268.   Try to get some psychological help. If you combine therapy with medication, it can help you deal with your depression. Therapy and medication together have proven to be more effective than either one is alone. Medication for depression can help avoid sudden drops in your mood, while a therapist can help you unravel and treat the causes of depression.

269.   A great tip that can help you out of your depression is to write your own poetry. Writing poetry can be very cathartic and therapeutic. Not only, will writing poetry help you get out of your depression, you'll also have a genuine work of art that you can be proud of.

270.   Do not be afraid to take your medication. Even if you do not think it is working for you sometimes it takes awhile for medication to build up in your system and begin working. Depression medication is not instant relief! Take it every day at the same time and give it a chance to do its job.

271.   Stave off depression by developing your interests. One of the prime factors in depression is a lack of interests and activities that you enjoy. Having an outlet for your interests contributes greatly to self-esteem and happiness. Doing things you enjoy, whether it is painting, hiking, reading, or volunteering keeps your mind off of your problems and gives great satisfaction.

272.   If you are suffering from depression, take a realistic account of your life now, as well as, your goals for the future. If you believe you 'can't be happy until' you have the ideal relationship, or higher income, or the like, then look at what is really important! Ask yourself if you "~it is really that bad now' or if you "~are setting reasonable goals.' If you are in a situation that is not likely to change, see if you can change the way you look at it.

273.   If you are depressed, it would be best for you not to hang around other depressed people. As the old saying goes, misery loves company. The last thing you need is someone rationalizing and promoting your misery. If you hang out with other depressed people, you will be down in the dumps forever, barring any kind of recovery.

274.   Just as you shouldn't be afraid to tell someone that you are suffering from clinical depression you also shouldn't feel obligated to tell everyone. If you are in a professional environment or any situation where you feel that others may not understand the severity of your situation, feel free to keep quiet.

275.   Try your hardest to maintain a healthy circle of friends and not just one best friend who you tell everything to. Your depression will cause even the best of friends to feel drained so it is essential that you spread these conversations out among several of your closest friends to even it out.

276.   You should never let yourself feel like a broken person because you are dealing with depression. Just as some people have to deal with bad lungs or a difficult disease, you have to deal with your depression. You should consider it to be nothing more than a nuisance in your life.

277.   Wear clothing that makes you feel happy. Your clothing should be a reflection of the mood you wish to be in, not the mood you are currently in. Wear something colorful and fun that will make you smile when you look at it.

Pick out your favorite outfit, even if it is formal, and wear it around the house to try to boost your spirits.

278.   A critical tip for anyone dealing with depression is to consciously realize when you are in need of professional assistance. Attempting to deal with serious cases of depression alone can lead to the escalation of the problem. Seeking medical or psychological help should never be a source of embarrassment, and can often lead to effective resolution of otherwise very thorny dilemmas.

279.   If you suffer from depression, it is important that you drink plenty of water. Medical research studies have shown that water can actually help to reduce depression symptoms. Try to have at least one glass of water before bed, to help you fall and stay asleep, and drink a glass in the morning.

280.   Refrain from seeking to be perfect. No one is perfect, regardless of the image they portray or the feelings they give off. Even with all the confidence in the world, perfection is a word for the Gods and you should always remember that you will have flaws, but it is these flaws that make you unique.

281.   To cure depression, you need to focus on being active. Exercise releases endorphins, which will naturally make you feel good. Don't think of this as a quick fix, but something you should be doing every day. If you think of being active as a life style, you will be much less likely to give up.

282.   Get a hobby. One of the most common reasons people develop depression is because they do not have enough interests to stay busy. Finding a hobby and developing an interest can help you to realize that you are good at something, and that others enjoy the same hobby that you do.

283.   A good tip that can help you get out of your depression is to start keeping a daily journal. Keeping a daily journal can be a good way to just get your feelings out and to express yourself honestly. You can also refer back to it if you want.

284.   Get exercise. Activity can be very therapeutic, so having a regular exercise schedules can make your life happier and healthier. Learning to enjoy your exercise and having a healthy life will cause you to increase your positive moods. Having proper nutrition

can also keep your health and happiness on a high note.

285.   A great tip that can help you beat depression, is to simply realize that depression doesn't last forever. It only lasts for a period of time. If you remind yourself of this, you can look through the fog to see the light. You have to realize that things will get better.

286.   Keep a journal. It is important to have an outlet for your feelings, as suppressing emotions is a key cause of depression in many people. If you do not have someone you are comfortable talking with, a journal makes the perfect listener. It does not judge, and can also serve as a reminder when you need to look back on your treatment.

287.   If you suffer from depression, having a pet can help alleviate this condition. Studies have shown that individuals who own pets are less likely to have depression. Having a pet will help you feel less isolated. Since pets need care, you will feel a sense of being needed. A feeling of being needed can be a powerful antidote to suffering from depression.

288.   Stop the bad and negative behavior when you are with others. Crying, complaining, and talking about your problems will elicit sympathy from your friends and family, but this sympathy also maintains the depressive behavior. Change the behavior and receive the rewards.

289.   Even if you have never felt depressed before in your life, that doesn't mean that it cannot start quickly and unexpectedly. Depression can have very late stage onsets so don't write it off even if you are in your forties or fifties. It can also strike both genders in almost equal amounts.

290.   If you are struggling with depression try not to get yourself caught up in the destructive mindset that the world is out to get you. This will only make you despair more and can do nothing but make your depression even worse and deeper than it was in the first place.

291.   Identify the reason for your depression! It can stem from a myriad of sources. Perhaps, it should be carefully analyzed by a professional. The most common causes of depression are circumstantial and clinical. Circumstantial is caused by difficult situations that are currently in the person's life, while clinical is caused by a chemical imbalance!

292.   Try to pamper yourself if your depression symptoms are bothering you. Going to a salon to have your nails done or going to a spa to have a massage can help relax your mind and body and thus, reduce your depression symptoms. You may also want to buy yourself a special treat, like a shirt you have been wanting.

293.   Music can help to fight depression, but keep in mind the kind of music you are listening to. Do not listen to music that engenders moody feelings of blues or melancholy. This music can make you dwell on your own feelings.

294.   If you are feeling depressed during the day try to stop what you are doing and go for a quick walk in the sun. Sunlight helps your body to release some chemicals that actually make you feel much happier. This is also true for people who are naturally depressed.

295.   One of the best things depressed people can do is to learn gratitude. Being thankful for the positive things that you have in your life, in comparison to those that are less fortunate, will make you appreciate what you have, instead of dwelling on the things that you don't have.

296.   Exercise. Studies have shown that people who exercise have lower rates of depression, and that those with depression can help their condition by doing some kind of exercise. Exercising is not only great for your physical health but for your mental health as well, so start an exercise program. There are many to choose from, and you'll feel much better.

297.   Keep a positive attitude. Negative thinking is always present in a person that has depression. Depressed people tend to minimize all of the good in their lives, while happy people keep a positive attitude by accepting sadness as a normal part of life, and fixing what they can. Being positive will also make you more pleasant to be around, and there is a lesser chance you will be lonely.

298.   When helping somebody else deal with depression, be sure that you are not an enabler of bad behavior. This is important because you will not help anybody by giving into behaviors that do not help the person recover. An example would be to allow the person to not eat dinner with you at the table and bring food to their room, or to allow them to remain in bed all day.

299.   Develop a method of reducing and preventing stress. Stress is a huge influence in your mood, causing depression when it gets too thick. If you are able to find a mental health center that can help alleviate your stress, you can find the right methods of alleviating depression as well as discover life to be a more positive experience when you aren't stressed out.

300.   A great tip that can help you out of your depression is to realize that making an effort to get better might make you uncomfortable. People will often stay depressed because it's comfortable. Attempting to fix your problems may be temporarily uncomfortable but it can lift you out of your depression.

301.   If you are feeling sluggish or lazy due to your depression and would like to feel more alert, you should think about introducing more protein into your diet. Foods such as soybeans, seeds, and lean meats have been shown to increase alertness and awareness and can be helpful for those days when you don't feel like getting up.

302.   If you are feeling depressed, and you have the means, consider adopting a pet. Even a small pet such as a rodent can give you the feeling that someone else depends on you each day. Having a

pet is especially helpful for beating depression if you live alone, since it means you don't come home to an empty house.

303.   Try to get outside as much as you can, when suffering from depression. Even if it is just for a quick walk every day, getting some sun and fresh air, can make a world of a difference for controlling depression symptoms. Sitting inside all the time, will just make you feel worse.

304.   Make sure that you understand all of the possible side effects before you decide to take any type of medication. Your doctor may be eager to prescribe you pills, and this may actually help you greatly, but you need to be sure that you are aware of exactly what you are taking ahead of time.

305.   Identify the reason for your depression! It can stem from a myriad of sources. Perhaps, it should be carefully analyzed by a professional. The most common causes of depression are circumstantial and clinical. Circumstantial is caused by difficult situations that are currently in the person's life, while clinical is caused by a chemical imbalance!

306.   Do not deny your emotions. For depression caused by a traumatic event or loss, it is important to let yourself feel the pain and sadness. You should not dwell on it, however, it is important to not bottle it away. It will only surface later, and often in more harmful ways.

307.   Keep your friends and family close. Many people are willing to help you deal with your depression. Allow them into your life and include them in your situation. You will be surprised how understanding people are. Connecting with others in any way will only be beneficial to you and they might even be able to provide a few smiles.

308.   If you have begun taking medication for depression, do not be alarmed if you do not feel better right away. In fact, you may even feel worse when your medication does not work because you are nervous. Most anti-depressants take at least three weeks to settle into your system and help your symptoms.

309.   Before you begin taking any medication for depression, do your homework and research the risks and benefits as well as any side effects. If one medication doesn't work, there are many to choose from, and your doctor will be happy to

experiment until you find one that has the least side effects and discomfort for you. Everyone reacts differently to a medication.

310.   For those who suffer from depression, get your spouse or partner to do the housework. It is important that you relax and avoid activities that could make your depression worse. If you feel bad about putting all of the responsibilities on to your spouse, offer to do the housecleaning one week and ask them to do it the next.

311.   An important way to deal with depression is to make sure that your goals and expectations are realistic. This is important because you are setting yourself up for further depression and disappointment if you are longing for something that is not possible. Be sure to share your wishes and desires to keep yourself in check.

312.   When it comes to dealing with depression, you may wish to consider listening to recordings that are of a motivational persuasion. This is important because a little coaching can sometimes be all that is needed in order to feel good about yourself. Check your local library for tapes before purchasing.

313.　Over indulging in food may seem to provide some immediate relief but in reality it will only lead to longer term disappointment and worsen depression. What ever is making you depressed will not be remedied by eating so try and find some other way to comfort yourself, one that you will not feel guilty about later.

314.　When it comes to dealing with depression, it is important to know what it is that can cause you to feel especially depressed. This is important because this is the first step to overcoming your issues - stopping the feelings from arising and eliminating what is causing you to feel this way.

315.　Get exercise. Activity can be very therapeutic, so having a regular exercise schedules can make your life happier and healthier. Learning to enjoy your exercise and having a healthy life will cause you to increase your positive moods. Having proper nutrition can also keep your health and happiness on a high note.

316.　Understand your mind. Depression is not a sign of insanity, rather it means something is not right. Depression is just a sign that something in your life is unbalanced. It could be something in yourself, your environment, or may include both. Knowing you are not crazy can really help you feel more positive about your life.

317.   Depression can seem never ending, but with the proper changes to your life, counseling and even medications if necessary, it will come to an end. You will emerge a happier and healthier you at some point. Keep your head up and try to think positively about the future. Above all, don't give up.

318.   Pretend that you are happy. Many times, putting a fake smile on, and attempting to act and think happily can actually cause your mood to change. Faking these changes with your body actually increases the amount of happiness-inducing chemicals produced, which causes you to start to feel the happiness you are outwardly portraying.